43 Days

43 Days

Born to live

Kimmy Littlejohn-Clark

XULON PRESS

Xulon Press
2301 Lucien Way #415
Maitland, FL 32751
407.339.4217
www.xulonpress.com

Unless otherwise indicated, Scripture quotations taken from the New King James Version (NKJV). Copyright © 1982 by Thomas Nelson, Inc. Used by permission. All rights reserved.

Scripture quotations taken from the Holman Christian Standard Bible (HCSB). Copyright © 1999, 2000, 2002, 2003, 2009 by Holman Bible Publishers, Nashville Tennessee. All rights reserved.

Paperback ISBN-13: 978-1-66280-707-7

Chapter 1

I'M PREGNANT!

I KNEW I WANTED TO BE A MOTHER FROM the time I was 16. I remember mommy said I had a "mothering spirit" because I always looked out for my twin Timmy. She would remind me periodically she was the mama.

My parents showed me what a Godly marriage looked like growing up. I'd say to myself when I grow up I'm gonna be a wife and mother. At 41 I was married and by 42 I was pregnant with my bundle. My body changed rapidly and I was thinking...I must be pregnant. I went to the doctor too soon and she told me I wasn't pregnant unless it had just happened. I told her oh it happened (lol) Later that night, I told my husband who was disappointed by the news I feel like I'm not alone. He said I'm right here. I said no, in my body I feel like I have company.

Let's rewind the story a little bit. Ok I told you that I knew I was gonna be a mother and when we decided to try my husband started to feel disappointed. I remember saying "oh yea of little faith". Now fast forward I found another doctor and learned my faith paid off. On December 7, 2011 I was already 2 months! My time had come so I rolled out my own red carpet and put on my tiara. I prayed for a baby and the Lord heard me. I couldn't thank the Lord enough...Chancz was on the way!

In my quiet time with the Lord I still sometimes wonder why it had to be this time in my life. I never imagined (and I do have a huge, crazy imagination) that I would be a mom/wife in my 40's. Nevertheless I was elated.

Chapter 2

LET THE JOURNEY BEGIN

I STILL SAY I HAD THE PERFECT PREG-
nancy in spite of my baby dying. I didn't have
hypertension or gestational diabetes. I was 42
years old and worked until I was 6 months. I look
back now and I see how the Lord was setting the
stage for what was to come. I went to the doctor
and she said you look tired Mrs Clark. I am gonna
write a note for you to be off. I felt like my energy
level was still high until after 6:30 pm. At that time
without fail I was ready to sleep.

Being home allowed me more time to just talk,
sing, and read psalm 121(I read it to him from
Dec 7, 2010- July26,2012) to Chancz. I was over
the moon happy and the Lord didn't allow nothing
to steal my joy. I recall a coworker saying to me
one day are you still believing you're gonna get

married and have a baby at 40? I said yes (thinking of Hebrew 11:1) she said girl I would've gave that dream up a long time ago. I said you said the right word "you would".

But, I'm not and I walked away laughing. When people mentioned my age I'd say what's your point?

Sarah was 90, now get off my red carpet. Read Genesis 17:15-19, Genesis 21:1-6

At my prenatal visits I began to hear he's growth restricted. There could be something wrong with his heart, but every time they turned on the monitor he had a strong heartbeat. They offered me the amniocentesis, but I declined. As the time went on they began to preach to me about doing tests and I finally said with much conviction NO!

I shared the story with them of Shadrach, Meshach and Abednego (Daniel 3). I said Look, I didn't get this old to lose faith now. Even if it is something wrong with my boy I am keeping him so stop asking. I loved on my baby more every day and couldn't wait to hold him. My main focus was to love on him and teach him about Jesus. I made a promise to the Lord and was determined to keep it. Numbers 30:2 and Ecclesiastes 5:4-5.

Chapter 3

FAITH WITHOUT WORKS

THE DOCTORS KEPT TELLING ME CHANCZ was growth restricted. I heard them, but I truly believe the Lord had me so overcome with joy that I was oblivious to what was really going on. I will always believe He allowed me to bask in my pregnancy because of the heartbreak ahead and for that I am beyond grateful. Everyone I came in contact with said I was one of the happiest pregnant women they'd seen. The joy of the Lord was indeed my strength (Nehemiah 8:10, Psalm 28:7).

I didn't think I was too good to experience trails, but now more than ever I had to exercise my faith. The Lord blessed my womb and I refused to let news from the doctors shake my faith. I do respect doctors and they had a job to do. So did I and this was my season (James 2:17). I read Psalm 121 so much Chancz should've come out quoting it. I told him Jesus would be his best friend (Proverb 18:24) . We both told him we loved him, but Jesus love him better than we could.

Chapter 4

LORD, WHAT'S GOING ON?

ONE SUNDAY AFTER CHURCH WE GRILLED and I noticed earlier that day Chancz didn't seem very active. He was always bouncing around. I felt the need to go to ER I told the family maybe he's supposed to slow down as I am in the last trimester. My husband said I simply ate too much. No sooner than they hooked up the monitors he started flipping. My bundle was Ok.i was like really boy? I thought maybe my husband was right. I had eaten too much and he was full and sleepy. As they discharged me I told the staff I feel so good I'm going home and eat my cold pineapples. And I think I'll just skip my appointment tomorrow and sleep in. They yelled, NO Mrs Clark never miss any appointments!

ABOUT MONDAY

Before I went to my appointment I noticed one of my ankles were swollen. I mentioned it to the nurse as soon as I arrived and said maybe my eyes were playing tricks on me as I felt tired. She said yes, it is swollen and took my blood pressure. I didn't notice how many times she took it until she took me to another room (I was on Facebook). Suddenly the doctor came in and said Mrs. Clark you've had good readings the entire pregnancy until today. We are admitting you now.

What? Can I at least go downstairs and get Chick Fil A? I promise I will come right back. What about my car? By the way for some reason everyone volunteered to go with me on this appointment and I said no. The one time I go alone and look what happened. I just broke down and cried. Then I prayed Lord, what's going on? Please help me understand. I am not ready.

Chapter 5

JUNE 13, 2012

I WAS GIVEN AN OPTION TO REMAIN PREG-nant for 7 weeks or deliver via C section. I'll take a C section for $200 please! The doctors told me he wasn't getting enough nutrients and he had stopped growing. She said to me (looking like she was only 20) I have a low tolerance for high blood pressure. Let me tell you, you won't be pregnant in July, or by the end of June. In fact if I could have it my way you wouldn't be pregnant by tonight. Mrs. Clark, you definitely won't be pregnant by the end of this week. Wow! My dear Chancz was deliv-ered...the room was quiet but I was still excited and exercising my faith. Everything will be Ok in spite of him coming now right?

I was floating from the medicine and still didn't know he was born sick until the next day. The doctor delivered the news like a pizza delivery only the delivery was bad and cold. He was born with Trisomy 18 and would die in a few days. She had a Santa Claus list of things wrong with him and talked so much I kid you not all I began to hear was blah blah blah. Would she ever stop adding to the list? I was in shock and when I went in his room I burst out crying. I felt like I was sleep walking or having a bad dream and when I woke up all would be Ok.

Chancz was on a ventilator with tubes everywhere. I had to wait a week to hold him I would go back to my room every night and cry and pray. I asked the Lord for a miracle. I asked the Lord Where will my faith lead me? As the days passed I gave myself pep talks and put my faith in full motion (Luke 17:6). I thanked the Lord daily for my boy. (1 Thessalonians 5:8, Ephesians 5:20). I said Lord I know what it looks like, but I'm gonna trust you. I remember saying I've got stupid faith (Hebrews 11:6) and my baby was a fighter. The Lord gave him enough strength to last 43 days. I pumped breast milk aka liquid gold.

So he was he was born at 2lbs 6 oz and reached 3 ½ lbs 6 oz total. I looked forward to seeing his face and would say Chancz, "mama's here". At night when I went home I would say see you later as I just knew I would get another day with him. I talked to him and sang Jesus loves the little children. I would read scripture and play gospel music for him. Doctors delivered bad news daily, but I was determined to keep my promise to the Lord... and that was teach him about Jesus (Ecclesiastes 5:5). The staff said wow, we've never seen a mother sing, pray and read the bible to her baby...you're amazing. I felt humbled and told them about my promise unto the Lord.

Chapter 6

REMEMBER TO GET BACK UP

MANY STORMS HAVE COME IN MY LIFE, BUT this one knocked me to the ground too hard. I felt like that commercial that's often shown on TV "I've fallen and I can't get up". When I came home late at night I felt I was on the floor mentally until the next time I saw my boy. It was up and down daily...I didn't want him to feel my sorrow so I smiled and held myself together. I felt so much hope when I looked at his innocent face (Isaiah 40:31) I haven't experienced pain like this ever. It feels like you're having a heart attack...the ache made me lose my breath. A woman who's lost a child knows exactly what I'm talking about.

The pain makes your heart ache under your skin literally. You carry a living soul for however long only to come home empty handed. Your stomach feels empty because your breakfast, lunch, and dinner buddy is no longer stealing your food or energy. When this happens the only one who can help you "get up" is Jesus Christ. If I didn't have a relationship with him Pre-Chancz I wouldn't be where I am today. When Chancz died I thought of Psalm 23:4....I must warn people when a parent loses a child they're never the same. We have to learn to find a new normal.. All of our dreams that are attached to Chancz died when he died (all mothers have dreams of what they will do with and for their child). We literally have to start from scratch. If you're in a relationship with Jesus all hope is not gone.

I serve Jesus and trust me He's the ultimate healer. I've been judged and misunderstood but I'm getting back up daily (and you know I returned the favor by judging back). One may call it being petty, well when it comes to my boy. IJS. Grieving parents I encourage you to find Jesus through your tragedy...the best time to invite him into your heart as Lord & Savior is now. He will calm the storm (Psalm 107:29). If your child loss is just beginning you may find it hard to believe what I'm saying. It's true you can get back up after child loss. I'm 6 yrs in, but I am up. Thank you Lord.

Chapter 7

WHAT'S WITH HIS NAME?

When my husband and I talked about having a baby I told him I already had a name. He loved it immediately.... We just had a tug of war on how it would be spelled (he won). He loved the name so much he said whether boy or girl that's the name. Honestly I wanted more kids, but as I got older that sorta changed.

Our former pastor came to pray for us before Chancz went to heaven and he said sister Clark I know you so I must ask what's the meaning behind his name?. I laughed and said yes pastor it is. I prayed and asked the Lord to give me one chance at a baby in my old age (40's) so when I found out I was pregnant that name felt perfect. We couldn't have chosen a better name for him. He came and even though his life was brief his life had a purpose.

He was on an assignment. When his assignment was up he left.

I felt his spirit lift up toward heaven as he took his last breath...what an experience. I've sat and ruminated about that day countless times. I reminded him about all the things I taught him about Jesus as (I rocked him for about 20 minutes) that he was going to heaven in a few minutes and Jesus would take care of him. I let him know Jesus would be his best friend. In my own spare time I let my spiritual imagination run wild and thought I wonder if Jesus said as he took his last breath come on my child it's time(and my baby's spirit surrendered). We all have to make sure when our name is called for death that Jesus is calling you to heaven and not eternal punishment (hell).

All of us will have an eternal home when the death angel comes. It's very important to know which place will be your final destination. My Chancz is home and one day I'll join him...that's why I never told him goodbye. I told him I will see him again that's why it was only necessary to say see you later my son. The doctor tried to put Chancz on a CPAP machine to see if he could go home to die. It was an epic fail so the hospital was his only earthly home. I had hoped he could come home on hospice, but the good Lord knew best. When the CPAP failed 5 minutes after they put him on it his body went limp and the Lord let me zoom in to his distress. That's when I knew Chancz wouldn't get an earthly healing.

The doctor looked and said what would you like to do? I said put him back on the ventilator, but we must let him go. Then I walked away as they hooked him back up. I cried and prayed... Lord I get it but if he has to go let me rock him to you. Then I walked over to his bed and said Chancz, Jesus loaned you to me for a little while, but you're gonna have to go. My boy opened his eyes and gave me a look like he understood. I'd like to think he was saying with his eyes Ok mama. I felt like he understood what I was saying to him. He really paid attention to us when we talked to him daily and he held onto our fingers tight. I can remember one time my husband had told him he was going downstairs or something and when he tried to let go of Chancz's finger he held on tight and pulled back. It was so precious and I can't be convinced he didn't have his own way of communicating with us. His little eyes said it all.

Chapter 8

PAYING BACK YOUR LOAN

WE ALL HAVE HAD SOME KIND OF LOAN IN our life that we've had to pay back. Have you ever had a heavenly loan? I have! The Lord deposited one in my womb. One would think if He deposits that kind of loan all we have to do is pay him back by training up a child right? I mean I am thinking as godly parent would possibly think (<u>Proverbs 22:6</u>). I learned there are other ways to pay a loan to the Lord. If I had known how bad the paid would be I think I may have asked to be taken to heaven myself instead. Abraham comes to mind when the Lord asked him to sacrifice his only son Isaac. In my own private thoughts I'm thinking Ok Lord you said he would be the father of many nations (<u>Genesis 17:1-5</u>). He then came back again and told him his wife would conceive in her old age (first of all they should've known the Lord was up to something. After all he changed their names then made them promises(Genesis 15-19. I can't blame Abraham or Sarah for laughing at that age, but the Lord showed himself mighty and most of all he kept his promise. I get excited because He is an awesome promise keeper no matter what.

The Christian journey is like none other. You will get weary, be afraid nevertheless the Lord says more than once in the bible "fear not" and "lo I am with you". Anyway, back to the outstanding loan I had to pay back...I had no idea he would expect me to pay him back by making me give my boy back to him after 43 days. The Lord gave me an amazing taste of motherhood, but every now and then I think of how much Job 1:21 applies to my life. I think of how Job 1:21 applied to my life. This was the hardest thing I have ever had to do. Children are gifts and parents ought to treat them as such. There's a popular saying motherhood is denied to many so I am forever grateful I was chosen to be Chancz's mama.

But lets talk about promises again for a minute. I promised to teach my baby about Jesus and like I said that would be one good way to pay the Lord.

Not many people realize that when one makes a promise to the Lord he expects us to keep it (Ecclesiastes 5:5). I took my promise seriously and was excited to get right on it even when I carried him. So I admonish people to think before making vow to the almighty God. He's too sovereign to be played with.

Parents if you ever feel ungrateful remember the Lord has no problem with fixing this issue. On the other hand he doesn't have to take your gift (child/children) from you. He can remove you from this equation and allow someone else to raise your child/children. Which would you prefer? This child loss journey is ongoing its also known as angel mommy life...regardless of the name it requires continuous healing from the day you pay your loan back until your last breath and/ or the rapture (when Jesus comes back to take his bride (all who have accepted him as lord and savior (Romans 10:9-10) back to heaven with him ! Thessalonians 5:16-18).

It's up to us to receive healing....its always available to a saint. Someone who doesn't live for the Lord doesn't realize how much the Lord is willing to heal. The word says he is close the brokenhearted

(Psalm 34:18). I've learned very quickly that not every grieving parent want healing because they may feel it will mean they are forgetting about their child. That's a myth, we never shall forget. On Chancz's death bed I made him a promise...i told him I would miss him every day until I joined him. Y'all already know this mama is keeping her word still 6 yrs later.

Time is precious so cherish it because one day it can be your turn to pay back a heavenly loan. Whether it's unexpectedly or you see the hand-writing on the wall ahead of time it hurts your heart so bad it leaves you breathless some days.

Chapter 9

UNANSWERED QUESTIONS

SINCE I ROCKED MY BABY TO HEAVEN ON July 26, 2012 I decided to call it 'Happy Heaven Day"! I celebrate it because of what the bible says in Ecclesiastes 7:1 I'm referring to the later part "and the day of death better than the day of birth" So I encourage parents to celebrate their child's life no matter how long or short their life was. It was a life. I have so many questions that remain unanswered such as I wonder how old my baby is in heaven? After all scripture says One day is like a thousand years (2Peter3;8). Does he take naps? Is there a heavenly playground? Are there toys up there? Does the Lord let him see me when I am tear-free? Does he remember all I taught him about Jesus when he was on earth? Does he still look like daddy?

All of these fall under the unanswered category. I'm not discouraged though, instead I'm to see how its all gonna turn out. My burning questions are Will he know I'm his mother? Will he call me mama? I love to daydream and smile about stuff like this. And the one thing I am sure about is one sweet day I will know all these answers. Parents you can find out these answers too if your name is written in the lambs book of life. Our baby's names were written in there long long ago (Rev 21:27). Mine was written in 1997. I am glad I was living for Jesus long before losing Chancz. I always tell people If I wasn't already living for Him Pre Chancz I'd have given up right after he died.

Chapter 10

DEAR CHANCZ

I STARTED A PAGE IN HIS MEMORY AFTER he died on FB to show other angel mommies its Ok to love on their babies out loud. I had no idea how many hid their love in fear of comments people would make. I tell you I learned the hard way how mean people can be after you lose a child...especially as the years roll on they expect you to really be over your child. There is no such thing.

I felt so much better because I feel healing when I write him love letters. I started before he died. On May 13, 2012

> Dear Chancz, I welcome you into the world and in my heart. So help me God I will teach you all I know about Jesus. I'm proud to be your mother

and want you to know you were conceived through a union called marriage. I don't regret having you later in life and pray that I see you become a man, a godly man. I want you to know Jesus is right now and in the future your best friend. I prayed for you and your salvation in advance and believe in faith it will happen. I wanted a 2 parent home for you so bad because I told God I want nothing less than what I had.

All I ask of you in return is to make me proud of you by being all that you can in other words do your best. And most importantly never be without the Lord. I recited Psalm 121 to you in my womb daily because you will need to be reminded of it throughout your entire life. Along with the rest of the bible so with that being said welcome

love mama

June 18, 2012

Dear Chancz, you are officially 5 days old now thanks to Jesus I'm home feeling so empty without you and don't know when the tears will end. I didn't get to see you til the next day and was overwhelmed by all the things going on. I said all of this to let you know even though a lot has happened you are alive, you are my strong boy. I love you very much and my heart went to pieces leaving you at the hospital on June 17, 2012. Please grow so you can come home. I don't want to be without you in this house for too long. I was very happy because you have so much life and color and I got to kiss you for the first time. You look like daddy. Anyway, just another love letter from my heart to you my son

As you can see I held on to my faith that he would come home and every day I counted and said yay…he made it again. It was a hope like none other.

June 21, 2102

Dear Chancz, you have been with us 8 days and yesterday was so good. Even though I didn't get to snuggle with you I m still so proud to be your mother and excited you had visitors. Pastor G came in and prayed over you. Daddy and I love you very much you give us a new meaning in life, you are bringing out the best in us. I can't wait for you to come home.

Love mama

One of my letters after he was gone:

June 13, 2012

Dear Chancz, happy birthday to you! I remember on so well I woke up in my right mind wanting to sing out loud but didn't instead I gave you the biggest shout out on Facebook. So many people chimed in on there. I got calls, texts and inboxed. I declare the Lord kept me from falling out I cried off and on but I made it. Aunt deb gave you the most beautiful shout out and she said the party you are having in heaven surpasses any day at Chuck e cheese. I'll never get to take you there, but its ok. I know where you are 24/7 and you're safe in Jesus arms

I dedicated "in the meantime" by BeBe and CeCe Winans to you

because I am gonna keep on loving
and missing you until I meet you in
heaven I love you forever my son

mama

I still write to him on his page but not as fre-
quently. I find some days I get off work and go and
go. Then it's bedtime and that's when I think of
him. It seems he's on my mind at night so heaven.
I say to myself this must be part of my angel
mommy journey.

Chapter 11

HE WAS BORN TO LIVE

MOST PARENTS WANT TO KNOW OR should I say all parents want to know why it had to be their child that had to die. And most believe its because they did something terrible in the past that made them feel unworthy to parent a living child. I can't lie I: felt all kinds of emotions and I wanted to know so I decided hey you know what? I'm in relationship with the Lord why not ask him? He will either tell me or he wont. So here goes. I prayed and said Lord, I waited my whole life and only asked for one child and you give him to me only to take him away. If its your will I want to know why he had to die. I kept praying Lord please tell me even if it hurts

2 years later I was sleeping and finally the Lord revealed to me that he didn't let him die to punish

me. He told me he let him die so he could use me to let people know (in particular angel mommies) who have lost their children that he is still worthy to be praised . He said I was his voice and I need to tell them to find Jesus though their tragedy. He didn't let him die to hurt me.

I am one of his representatives sharing my story and encouraging parents life isn't over. In fact it can began again in and with him. Romans 10; 9, 2 Corinthians 5;17. I must not sit down on the Lord and not help some angel parents whose heart aches like no tomorrow. I am gonna speak until I am no more because someone is willing to listen. I dare not believe that some parent is gonna give their life to Jesus just by reading this. I have come too far not to keep going. I don't know what the future hold but I tell you what this angel mommy is gonna keep walking with Jesus til the bitter end. I simply admonish you don't throw in the towel. Let your new normal without your child begin with Jesus.

Chapter 12

SO HAPPY FOR YOU BUT

Every time I hear someone is pregnant (especially someone I know) I really do feel happy for them. I just began to feel so much sorrow for myself. Then immediately I follow their pregnancy and write in my own head "and their baby was born and lived happily ever after. I'm almost willing to bet I am not the only angel mommy who writes another mother's story. The bottom line is I want every mother to get to the finish line and leave the hospital with hands that are full.

Nothing is worse than having a baby and walking out those doors with an empty womb and hands. Even so no matter how brief life is every life is precious and matters. My time with Chancz is frozen ...pictures, special milestones, birthdays etc is frozen. Or should I say on "pause"....hmmm maybe I will say the latter because his heavenly life is nowhere near frozen. He is growing up with Jesus! WOW, that makes my heart leap. I think I am at a point where I really understand(years later) can see how that scripture all things work together for the good of them who love God...y'all know the rest(Romans 8 :28). I honestly think as time goes on I am gonna keep learning more about how this angel mommy journey goes. I couldn't plan for such a tragedy and still sometimes feel when I go to bed at night that this was just a dream. Then I realize I have survived once again and that I will keep pressing on. I want to go on because the Lord has helped me find my "new normal" and I always end up smiling after every tear I shed.. A friendly reminder to all angel moms....in particular christian moms. Healing is continuous and available at all times of day and night. It's up to us to cry to the Lord for help. The Lord hears us (Psalm 18:6).

Chapter 13

TRIGGERS

You never know when there will be a trigger or should a say a wave of sorrow. They will come as your angel mommy journey goes on. There is no time to prepare for the waves...it can happen so fast you say wait a minute I was just laughing now I am crying a river! Since Chancz has been gone some days I can feel a wave and I either succumb to it and get my ugly cry on then there are some days I just don't want to cry.

Every time I cry the Holy Spirit comes to my rescue and soothes my achy heart....I am truly grateful because it literally feels like someone is rubbing my heart. What a feeling! I cry tears of sorrow because I miss him dearly. I sometimes babysit and when the children leave the house is too quiet...one time I had to get in my car and ended up at a store just to hear noise. Quiet moments with the Lord is way better than too much quiet after children leave your home. If you're not an angel parent you wouldn't understand. Be grateful you don't.

Maybe parents who are just experiencing what's called "empty nest" may come close to feeling what I feel. I may ask some empty nesters what their experience is like. Well I've said all this to say don't hold in your grief to make someone else feel comfortable. It will only make you more miserable in the end. Don't be afraid to love on your child out loud...it's a good way to feel some healing. I found myself holding back with my friends and this one angel mommy liberated me. She said if they're really your friends they will listen to you talk about your dead baby as you listen to them talk about their living children. From that day on I stopped holding back. This really is a two way street thing here...just because people have living children doesn't mean an angel mommy can't get tired of hearing stories about them. I think of Eve when Abel was killed by his own brother(Genesis 4:8). The Lord allowed her to be soothed in some way by blessing her and Adam with another baby.

Genesis 4:17. The world refers to it as having a "rainbow baby" (a baby born after the loss of one).

I am getting older, but still believe it can happen for me too. I always am excited to see what the Lord has up his Holy sleeve.

My story is not all sad, it has such a message for all who choose to learn from it. Chancz taught me a lot in such a short time…as I said before he was on assignment and helped me to remember I am on one too for the Lord. I plan on working mine until I hear the Lord call my name. In the meantime my prayer is:

Father in Heaven, I pray you touch the hearts of the one who take the time to read this book. May it encourage them like never before to keep going on. May they find your precious son Jesus through their loss and surrender their hearts unto salvation in the name of Jesus I ask it all Amen.

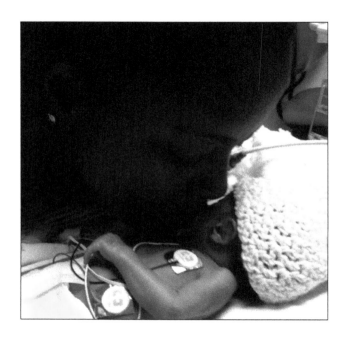

CPSIA information can be obtained
at www.ICGtesting.com
Printed in the USA
BVHW091419160221
600149BV00005BA/168